SKILLS UPDATE

BOOK 3

ILLUSTRATED BY MIKE BOSTOCK

Edited by
Sue Smith, Editor,
Community Outlook

Designed by
Hilary Tranter

First edition 1994
Reprinted 1995
Reprinted 1996

Published by
Macmillan Magazines Ltd
Porters South
Crinan Street
London N1 9XW

Printed in Great Britain by Pro Litho, London

ISBN 0-333-62296-0

FOREWORD

As the move towards care in the community progresses, more and more people require both holistic health care and a wide range of technical nursing procedures in their own homes.

Early hospital discharge, day surgery and out-patient treatments mean that early post-operative care such as pain relief and bowel care is increasingly becoming the responsibility of nurses working in the community.

Skills Update 3, the third collection of articles from the popular series which appears each month in *Community Outlook*, is intended to give nurses and students an understanding of a range of procedures, such as peritoneal dialysis and tracheostomy care, affecting their patients and clients in the community.

It is not intended to be a first-line teaching series for new skills but, rather, to be used as an update to encourage practitioners to reflect on skills they may have learned some time ago or to provide background information and an overview of technical procedures experienced by patients so that the best holistic care can be given, whatever the patient's environment.

Increasing use of skill mix for the delivery of care to people at home and in residential care means that a wider range of carers need education about the care of people who may previously have received more nursing input — for example, people who have a plaster cast or who need an orthosis.

The Skills Update books may prove useful as aids to those who are teaching non-nurse carers about treatments their relatives or clients are receiving.

It is hoped that the books will be used as a basis for discussion between nurses, students and clinical specialists in hospitals and residential care as well as in general practice and in the community.

Sue Smith
Editor, *Community Outlook*

CONTENTS

WHAT IS AN ORTHOSIS?

An orthosis is an external appliance used when there is need for support or realignment of limbs, joints or spine. Orthoses include splints, calipers, braces, harnesses, collars, corsets, footwear and shoe adaptations. A prosthesis is a replacement for a bodily part, that is, a hip or knee joint replacement, a false eye or breast, a hearing aid or artificial limb.

REASONS FOR ORTHOSES

Active treatment
- Splints to immobilise fractures or dislocations
- Harnesses or splints to correct congenital hip dislocation
- Braces to control the deformity of scoliosis
- Calipers to relieve weight from the hip in Perthes' disease

To maintain correct positioning
- A means of support for arthritic joints or spastic limbs
- Boots to retain position following correction of club foot
- Knee or shoulder brace to retain joint position

To provide support and limit movement to ease pain
- Supportive collar following neck injury
- Joint support after injury or surgery
- Lumbar corset for low back pain

To compensate for a disability
- A drop foot splint
- A cock-up splint for drop wrist

To ensure stability for weakened areas
- A leg splint in cerebral palsy
- A soft collar for rheumatoid arthritis of the neck

To assist movement and activity
- A working splint in limb nerve paralysis
- A toe-raising splint to assist ankle dorsiflexion
- A walking brace for those with paraplegia

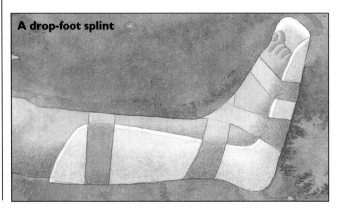

A drop-foot splint

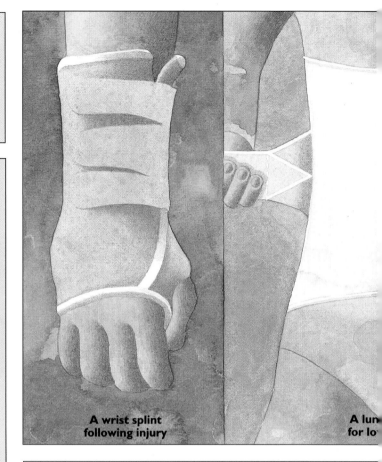

A wrist splint following injury

A lun for lo

SOLVIN

For a number of reasons, clients may choose not to persist with use of the prescribed orthosis and the nurse must ascertain why this has happened.
- The orthosis may be worn during the daytime, at night-time, all the time, periodically, during activity, when in pain, when standing or walking. In the early stages, there may be discomfort, but generally should be comfortable to wear. Tolerance may be achieved by sho periods of wearing the appliance and increasing the time span gradually.
- Does the client understand why he or she has been given the orthosis, its purpose and its mode of action and how to take care of it?
- Does the client find the orthosis stigmatising? If the client feels it is unsightly or attracts undue attention, this may discourage effective use, expecially in teenagers. Discuss ways of making the orthosis more unobtrusive and inconspicuous; cover with a glove or sock o conventional bandage, loose trousers, a large T-shirt or high-necke sweater or outdoor cape.
- Observe the skin for redness, irritation, burning or sore areas. Be alert to any rash that may indicate an allergic reaction to the orthotic material or result from sweat collecting. It is advisable to

ORTHOSES

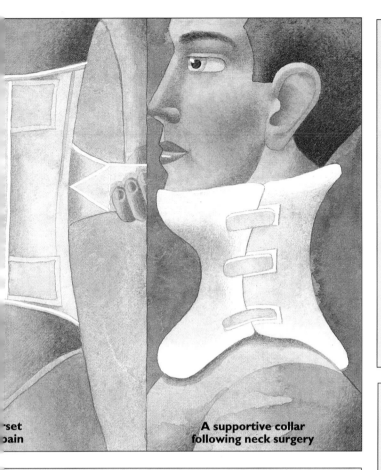

**set
pain**

**A supportive collar
following neck surgery**

ORTHOSIS CHECKLIST

■ Is the orthosis providing active treatment, preventing deformity, aiding mobility or relieving pain? Has the problem been resolved? If so, seek advice as to whether the orthosis may be discarded.

■ The orthosis should be handled with care and examined for cracks, chips, areas of wear or damage that may need attention to prevent chafing the skin. Is a new one or larger version required?

■ The fit may need adjusting if the client loses or gains weight or if swelling occurs or recedes in a limb. Children may need progressive serial orthoses to match their growth. If too tight, the orthosis will cause skin indentation and pressure, perhaps leading to neurovascular impairment, indicated by throbbing, aching, swelling, tingling or a pins-and-needles sensation in the limb. If too loose, it will cause skin irritation from friction and will fail to offer adequate support.

■ The viability of fastenings and straps should be checked. Is any padding wearing thin or fraying? Do edges need trimming? Does the client know how to care for the orthosis — cleaning, wiping, drying, oiling moving parts?

NOW YOU SHOULD FEEL COMPETENT TO:

■ Offer advice and support to clients and carers in the management of orthoses

■ Know what to observe for and when to refer the client back to the orthotist or specialist department.

FURTHER READING
Stewart, J., Hallet, J. *Traction and Orthopaedic Appliances.* Edinburgh: Churchill Livingstone, 1983.
Footner, A. *Orthopaedic Nursing.* London: Baillière Tindall, 1992.

Irene Heywood Jones, SRN, RMN, ONC, DipN, RNT, is a nurse tutor in orthopaedics and elderly care at St Vincent's Hospital, Pinner, and a freelance writer

OBLEMS

move the skin under the orthosis at regular intervals to relieve pressure and limit build-up of moisture. Special care is needed with the skin of infants, elderly people and clients with rheumatoid arthritis who are prone to fragile papery skin and nodule formation. Ensure the client can manage general personal hygiene. Skin under the orthosis must be kept clean and perfectly dry with a very light dusting of powder. Parents will need precise instructions on bathing and nappy application for an infant with a brace for congenital dislocation of the hip or a scoliosis brace. Clients with orthoses for back and neck problems will need advice on bathing and washing the hair.

Ensure that the client knows how to exercise the unsplinted limb and joints to retain his or her strength and power and can pursue activities for independent living as near normal within the limitations of the orthosis.

Clients may encounter difficulty in putting the orthosis on and taking it off. If they have hand weakness or problems with manual dexterity, have difficulty bending, are frail, unsteady, visually impaired or have cognitive impairment or learning disability, it may be necessary to involve a carer with orthosis management instructions and demonstration.

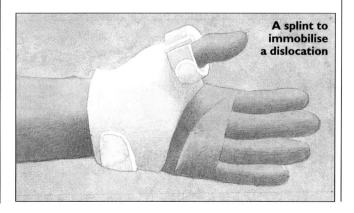

**A splint to
immobilise
a dislocation**

NASOGAST

WHO WILL PRESENT?

- Patients unable to ingest an adequate balanced diet orally. Nasogastric feeding is an effective method of providing supplementary or total nutritional support.

INDICATIONS

- Obstruction in the upper gastrointestinal tract which prevents normal ingestion, such as in oesophageal carcinoma or stricture.
- Cases of dysphagia caused by such conditions as motor neurone disease or cerebral tumours, where the quality of life is otherwise good.
- Cases of fistula when food taken orally may be aspirated.
- To improve overall nutritional status when a patient is too weak to take adequate calories by mouth.
- In conditions where discomfort or ulceration affects eating, for example, after facial surgery and during radiotherapy.

SAFE PRACTICE

- It is essential to ensure the tube is actually in the stomach before beginning each feed. There are three ways this may be done:
  - Aspirate some material and test its acidity using litmus paper; the hydrochloric acid in the stomach will turn blue litmus paper red
  - Inject 5ml of air down the tube while listening over the stomach with a stethoscope; a characteristic 'rumbling' sound should be heard
  - If it is felt necessary radio-opaque tubes may be checked using X-ray; this may be particularly relevant in cases where a fistula is present.
- If any change is observed in the patient's respiratory status during feeding, the feed should be stopped at once and the position of the tube rechecked.

ASPECTS TO CONSIDER IN ENTERAL NUTRITION

- If all the diet is taken via the nasogastric route, dietetic advice should be taken and the patient's condition should be assessed regularly.
- Nutritional status may be monitored by recording intake and by regular monitoring of weight. Other body measurements may also be recorded such as skin-fold thickness and upper arm circumference (so-called anthropometric measurements).
- Tolerance to therapy should be monitored. This should include observation and recording of nausea and vomiting, diarrhoea or constipation. The nurse should be ready to discuss the patient's feelings about nasogastric feeding and be aware of the psychological effects.
- Vitamin and mineral status should always be considered.
- Blood chemistry may be monitored for urea, electrolytes and glucose, and the urine tested for blood and glucose.

MANAGEMENT PRINCIPLES

- Pay attention to oral, nasal and skin hygiene. Tubes may chafe on the nasal vestibule (the front part of the nasal cavity which contain hairs) causing skin infection and possible ulceration. This area should be inspected and cleaned regularly. Vaseline may be applied for the patient's comfort.
- Excessive crusting within the nose which may complicate facial radiotherapy can be softened with 25% glucose in glycerol drops eight-hourly. Secretions and crusts can then be loosened with steam inhalations.
- Poor oral hygiene may result in mouth infections, so it is important to keep the mouth moist. Regular mouthwashes and care of teeth and dentures will help to moisten the mouth and reduce the build-up of debris. Oral hydration may be aided by use of artificial saliva and by sucking ice cubes. Vaseline may be used to keep the lips moist.
- The tube should be secured to the side of the face using a light tape. This should be done as unobtrusively as possible, particularly when the patient wants to leave the house. The end of the tube can be tucked over and behind the ear.
- Both patients and carers should understand the management principles of feeding and how to get supplies of feeds. Pharmacists and enteral feed-producing companies will normally deliver feeds directly to the home. Most manufacturers also employ a pump loan scheme.
- Eating is a social and emotional experience as well as a physiological necessity. For this reason it may help if a patient can have feeds at about the same time the family takes a meal. This promotes the normal social interaction of mealtimes.
- Some patients benefit from chewing, tasting and spitting out normal food. This may alleviate feelings of food deprivation.

ADMINISTRATION OF FEEDS

- Feeds may be given by interrupted bolus or by controlled continuous drip using gravity or pump.
- Bolus feeding is usually more convenient in the community because the patient spends less time connected to the feeding system. Feeding regimes can be tailored to an individual's lifestyle, permitting freedom of movement between meals.
- A regime should be monitored carefully. If it is not compatible with an individual, symptoms such as nausea, vomiting, abdominal distension and discomfort may result.
- Gravity feeding can limit mobility within the home as the feeding container must always be above the patient.
- Undesirable side-effects may be minimised and absorption maximised by using a pump-controlled infusion. If this is restrictive, feeds may be administered overnight.

IC FEEDING

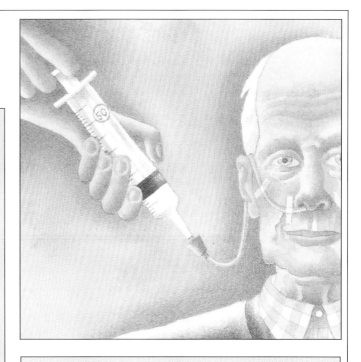

ADMINISTRATION OF BOLUS FEEDS

■ The temperature at which a tube feed may be administered varies. Administration of cold feeds has only a minimal effect on gastric emptying. Bolus feeds should be given at approximately 37°C.
■ The tube position should be checked to ensure it is in the stomach.
■ The feed may be run in by gravity or a 50ml syringe used to apply gentle pressure to push the feed into the stomach.
■ After feeding, the tube should be rinsed through with water to prevent stasis of feed in the tube which could cause infection.
■ Spigot the tube after the feed.
■ Drugs should not be mixed with the feed but given separately. Where possible, drugs should be given in aqueous solutions.
■ Tubes may be left *in situ* for several months before they need to be changed.
■ If the tube becomes blocked or does not seem to be in the stomach the tube should be replaced. If radiological checking is required the patient should be referred back to the hospital.

PROBLEMS AND SOLUTIONS

■ Nausea and vomiting:
— Give smaller feeds and consider using anti-emetics.
■ Gastric reflux and aspiration:
— Feed with the patient in an upright position
— Avoid night feeds
— Check residual volumes in the stomach before feeding; if these exceed 75–100ml then reassess feed volumes.
■ Constipation:
— Introduce a fibre-containing feed and ensure adequate systemic hydration. Encourage patient mobility. If these measures fail, consider laxative use.
■ Diarrhoea:
— Causes may include infection and antibiotic use
— Feed volumes may be reduced
— Intestinal osmolarity may be reduced by use of isotonic feeds
— Lactose-free feeds may be tried
— Pectin may be added to the feed
— Anti-diarrhoeal medication may be considered if other measures fail.

NOW YOU SHOULD BE ABLE TO:

■ Assess the needs of patients requiring nasogastric feeds
■ Recognise possible complications associated with tube feeding and suggest remedies.

FURTHER READING
Holmes, S. Enteral feeding. *Community Outlook* 1992; **2**: 10, 15–18.
Pritchard, A.P., David, J.A. *Manual of Clinical Nursing Procedures*. London: Harper and Row, 1988.
Saunders, E.H., Havener, W.H., Carol, F.K., Gail, H. *Nursing Care in Eye, Ear, Nose and Throat Disorders*. St Louis, Missouri: C.V. Mosby, 1979.

John Campbell, BA, RMN, RGN, DipN, CertEd, is nurse tutor, Lakeland College, Cumberland Infirmary, Carlisle

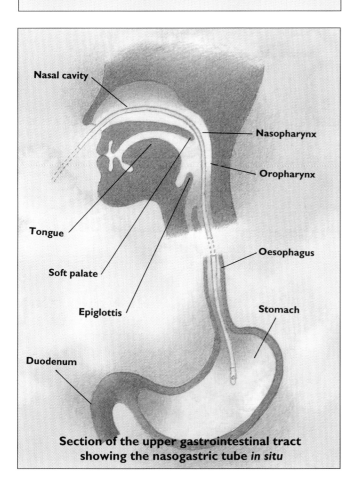

Nasal cavity

Nasopharynx

Oropharynx

Tongue

Soft palate

Oesophagus

Epiglottis

Stomach

Duodenum

Section of the upper gastrointestinal tract showing the nasogastric tube *in situ*

SUPPOS

WHO MAY PRESENT?

- Patients whose medication has been prescribed in suppository form. Some drugs are efficiently absorbed through the rectal mucosa. Drugs commonly given by this route include prochlorperazine, metronidazole and indomethacin. Aminophylline suppositories are no longer licensed because of erratic absorption and proctitis.[1]
- Patients requiring bowel evacuation prior to X-ray or bowel investigations as out-patients, for example, using Dulcolax suppositories
- Patients whose constipation has been assessed and for whom suppositories are the prescribed treatment. This may now be more common in the community as nurses provide general post-operative bowel care following day surgery and earlier hospital discharge.

CONTRA-INDICATIONS

- Suppositories and enemas should not be given in cases of rectal bleeding, colonic obstruction, paralytic ileus or following gynaecological or gastrointestinal surgery until the cause of constipation has been established and/or suppositories are medically prescribed.

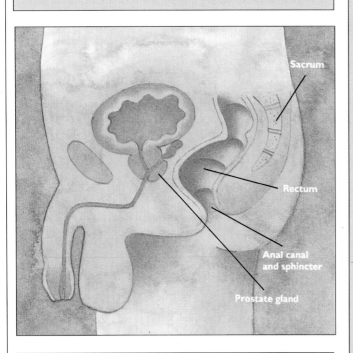

EQUIPMENT REQUIRED

- Tray
- Suppositories
- Clean gauze swabs or tissues
- Disposable gloves
- Water-soluble lubricant
- Clinical waste bag
- Protective covering for the bed
- Disposable apron
- Toilet, bedpan or commode

ADMINISTRATIO

- Gaining the patient's cooperation is important so that he or she will able to relax the rectal sphincter muscles in order to allow entry int the rectum.
- Close observation of the patient's overall condition is vital throughou the procedure, as vagal stimulation can cause vasodilation and bradycardia. For the same reason the whole procedure must be carried out as gently as possible. With gentle technique vasovagal reactions are very rare.
- Patient privacy must be ensured and interruptions avoided. This will also help the individual to relax.
- The patient should lie on his or her left side. In this position the rectu and colon slope downward allowing gravity to aid the entry of mater The knees may be bent up to improve patient stability and to aid exposure of the anus.
- A protective covering may be placed under the patient's buttocks an sheet positioned over the patient to minimise exposure.
- Suppositories may be removed from their wrapping and kept on a piece of clean gauze. The end to be inserted first should be covered with a water-soluble lubricant. This reduces friction as the supposito passes through the anus.

INSERTION OF SUPPOSITO

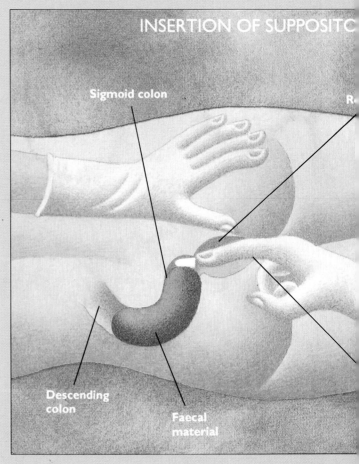

TORIES

F SUPPOSITORIES

To promote defecation the suppositories should be introduced with the pointed, thicker end first.

It has been suggested that if a systemic drug is being given per rectum the thin, flat end should be inserted first.[2]

The buttocks are parted using the left hand (in a right-handed practitioner). The patient is asked to take deep breaths through the mouth and to relax his or her anal sphincter. The suppository is inserted through the anus, then gently pushed along as far as possible using the index finger.

If the suppository contains a medication to be absorbed it should be positioned next to the rectal mucosal wall and not pushed into a faecal mass. In this case, if the rectum is loaded, an attempt to evacuate the mass should precede the administration of medication.

The anal area is wiped and the patient advised to retain the suppositories for as long as possible. The patient should remain on his or her side for five minutes after insertion to prevent premature evacuation. Access to a commode or toilet should be convenient.

All equipment should be hygienically disposed of. Gloves should be turned inside out during removal to prevent possible cross-infection. The result of the procedure should be observed and recorded.

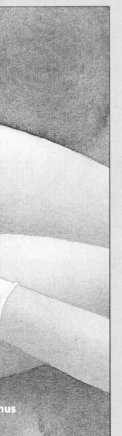

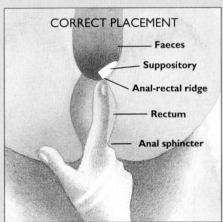

CORRECT PLACEMENT

- Faeces
- Suppository
- Anal-rectal ridge
- Rectum
- Anal sphincter

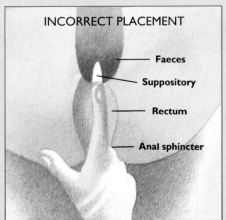

INCORRECT PLACEMENT

- Faeces
- Suppository
- Rectum
- Anal sphincter

nus

CONSTIPATION

■ Although constipation is more common in elderly people, because of their reduced mobility and poor appetite, it may occur at any age.

■ There is no 'normal' frequency of bowel movements, but individuals are usually aware of a reduction in the norm for them.

■ Many drugs have a constipating side-effect, for example, those used in Parkinson's disease, as well as many analgesics, especially codeine or opiate-based drugs, and appropriate preventive advice should be given.

■ Apathy and immobility are a major cause of constipation for many community patients. Those suffering from dementia may not be able to concentrate long enough to sit on the lavatory for a bowel movement.

■ It should be remembered that a change in bowel habit and a feeling of fullness after defecation are possible symptoms of colonic malignancy. In this case stools should be tested for occult blood and a medical opinion sought.

■ The essential components in prevention of constipation are fibre and fluids. If a high-fibre diet is taken with inadequate fluids the dry fibre may cause constipation. Ideally the diet should contain both water- and non-water-soluble fibre. Water-soluble fibre is found in fruit, vegetables and oats. Cereal products such as wholemeal bread and rice are rich in non-water-soluble fibre.

■ Active exercise should be encouraged as this increases peristalsis.

■ All treatments should be accompanied by dietetic advice to prevent recurrence of the problem. Changes in diet and life-style should be tried first. Laxatives, suppositories and enemas should be used as a last resort unless straining is exacerbating conditions such as angina or increases the risk of rectal bleeding as with haemorrhoids.

YOU SHOULD NOW BE ABLE TO:

■ Assess the need for suppository administration
■ Decide when medical referral is indicated
■ Be aware of the correct way to insert suppositories according to their purpose
■ Give health education on the prevention of constipation.

REFERENCES
[1] Clinical Pharmacy. *Pharmaceutical Journal* 1990; **244**: 659, 764.
[2] Pritchard, A.P., David, J.A. (eds). *Royal Marsden Manual of Clinical Nursing Procedures* (2nd edn). London: Harper and Row, 1988.

FURTHER READING
Hopkins, S.J. *Drugs and Pharmacology for Nurses* (11th edn). Edinburgh: Churchill Livingstone, 1992.
Perry, A., Potter, P.A. *Pocket Nurses' Guide to Basic Skills and Procedure.* St Louis, Missouri: C.V. Mosby, 1986.
Smith, F., Ross, F. Laxatives. *Community Outlook* 1992; **2**: 11, 21–24.
Turner, A. Constipation and faecal incontinence. *Professional Nurse* 1987; **2**: 8, 256–260.

John Campbell, BA, RMN, RGN, DipN, CertEd, is nurse tutor, Lakeland College, Cumberland Infirmary, Carlisle

INDICATIONS

- Most commonly, individuals who suffer from chronic renal failure will require peritoneal dialysis.

- Others include those who are unable to tolerate haemodialysis or those who have opted for peritoneal dialysis.

BACKGROUND ANATOMY AND PHYSIOLOGY

- The peritoneal cavity is a closed sac composed of serous membrane.
- The peritoneal membrane consists of two layers: the outer parietal layer lines the abdominal wall and the inner visceral layer covers the organs in the abdominal and pelvic cavities.
- The parietal and visceral layers are in contact and lubricated by a serous fluid, so normally the cavity is only a potential one.

- With a large surface area and a good blood supply the peritoneum acts as a dialysing membrane, molecules transferring from an area of high to an area of lower concentration.
- Although dialysis substitutes for the excretory functions of the kidneys, it does not replace the endocrine and homeostatic functions. It is for this reason that people on dialysis frequently suffer from bone demineralisation and anaemia.

THE PERITONEAL DIALYSIS CYCLE

Dialysis involves three stages, inflow, dwell and drainage through a peritoneal catheter which remains *in situ*.
- Inflow involves the infusion of the dialysis solution at body temperature into the peritoneal cavity.
- During dwell time the solution is left in the peritoneal cavity. Toxins and fluid in the blood will transfer out into the solution until the equilibrium point is reached.
- The peritoneal cavity is then drained to remove the solution, along with the toxins from the body.

CHOICE OF SOLUTION

- A solution protocol will be prescribed by medical staff. However, patients may be taught to vary the solutions if they find themselves becoming over- or under-hydrated.
- Dialysis fluids contain different concentrations of dextrose; the higher the concentration the more water is transferred from the blood into the solution by osmosis. The most common concentrations of dextrose are 1.36%, 2.27% and 3.86%.

METHODS OF DIALYSIS

Dialysis may be intermittent or continuous.
- Intermittent peritoneal dialysis is often carried out in hospital.
- Continuous ambulatory peritoneal dialysis is an effective self-care home treatment for chronic renal failure. The individual is free to walk around and perform most normal activities. It is a continuous process usually involving four exchanges per day, the last infusion remaining in the peritoneal cavity overnight.

  Various systems are in use and manufacturers' instructions should be consulted. If a 'Y'-type system is used, each cycle consists of connecting the tubing to the peritoneal catheter and running out the used solution. This outflow usually takes about 20 minutes. Then the new solution is run into the peritoneum. The tubing is disconnected and the patient left with only the peritoneal catheter *in situ*. The end of the catheter is closed and a new cap used as a cover every time. The dwell period is four to six hours.
- Automated peritoneal dialysis uses a machine to facilitate the cycles. It may be intermittent or continuous.

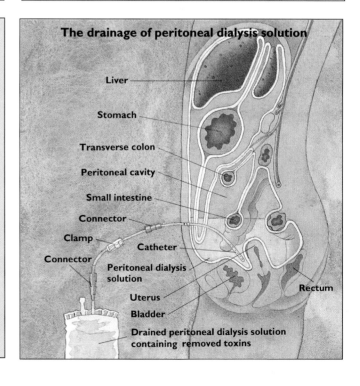

The drainage of peritoneal dialysis solution

Liver

Stomach

Transverse colon

Peritoneal cavity

Small intestine

Connector

Clamp

Connector

Catheter

Peritoneal dialysis solution

Uterus

Bladder

Rectum

Drained peritoneal dialysis solution containing removed toxins

MANAGEMENT

- Maintenance of aseptic technique is vital to prevent peritonitis.
- While the patient is adjusting to treatment, recordings of pulse, blood pressure and temperature may be carried out.
- Drugs such as heparin or antibiotics may be added to the dialysis solution.
- Iodine connection shields are used to prevent contamination entering at the tube junctions.
- After outflow of the previous solution, the bag of dialysis solution is attached to the giving set. It is allowed to flow into the peritoneal cavity by gravity. Typically, two litres of fluid will be used per cycle.
- The volume drained is recorded and compared with the volume infused.
- Regular assessment should be made of the effectiveness of the dialysis, a weight chart should be kept and occasional blood chemistry assessment performed.
- Nurses must take all the usual essential precautions employed when dealing with a body fluid.

POTENTIAL PROBLEMS

- The drained solution should always be observed for clouding, which indicates peritonitis. If this occurs, immediate medical help should be sought.
- Any indication of fever, feelings of abdominal fullness, persistent abdominal pain, cramps or unduly slow drainage may also indicate peritonitis. Antibiotics will be prescribed and given in the dialysis solution.
- Signs of fluid overload include systemic oedema, shortness of breath (caused by pulmonary oedema), chest pain, hypertension, headache, puffiness around the eyes and sudden weight gain.
- Excess fluid loss may be recognised by dizziness, postural hypotension, nausea, sudden weight loss, muscular cramps, thirst and dry mouth.
- If overload is occurring it indicates that the dialysis fluid is too dilute. Dehydration may result from a solution which is too hypertonic (that is, too high in dextrose). A change in the fluid regime may be indicated.
- Oral fluids should be encouraged in dehydration but restricted in overload.
- The catheter exit site should be monitored for signs of inflammation or infection and medical advice sought.
- If dialysis fluid leaks, bypassing the catheter, medical advice should be sought. If the catheter has to be changed, the patient will need to be admitted to hospital.
- The patient's body image can be damaged by the invasive nature of the treatment, and sexual difficulties may arise.
- Difficulties may arise when employers do not understand the constraints of the treatment regime.

PATIENT EDUCATION

- Asepsis must be maintained, especially when changing bags. The patient must know the principles and practice of aseptic technique. A clean working area should be set aside in the home if at all possible.
- The patient must know how to recognise early signs of peritonitis.
- The patient must understand the solutions used and how often exchanges are required.
- The importance of regular weighing should be clearly explained because of the implications of under- or over-hydration.
- Exit-wound care should be explained and dressing techniques taught.
- The patient may be supplied with a 'flat plate' to warm the bags of solution. Bags should never be warmed in a microwave and warming in hot water should be discouraged.
- Supplies of materials and fluids are usually delivered to the home by the manufacturers. Liaison with and visits by a specialist dialysis nurse should be arranged and encouraged.
- Advice should be sought from the dietitian and reinforced by the nurse. It is important to ensure that patients are well nourished and are getting enough protein. Studies have shown that a low albumin level significantly increases mortality rates in patients who are undergoing peritoneal dialysis.[1]

NOW YOU SHOULD BE AWARE OF

- The rationale for treatment by intermittent or continuous peritoneal dialysis
- The nursing skills involved in home continuous ambulatory peritoneal dialysis
- The patient's role in self-care and the nurse's role in providing support and education to both the patient and his or her family
- The need for early identification of potential problems.

REFERENCE
1. Parker, T.F., Laird, M.N., Lowrie, E.G. Comparison of study groups with NCDS and a description of mortality. *Kidney International* 1983; 23 (suppl.): S42–49.

FURTHER READING
Bloe, C.G. Peritoneal dialysis. *Professional Nurse* 1990; 5: 345–349.
Jerrum, C. CAPD: the state of the art. *Nursing* 1991; 4: 28–30.

John Campbell, BA, RMN, RGN, DipN, CertEd, is nurse tutor, Lakeland College, Cumberland Infirmary, Carlisle

RESUSCITATION

WHO MAY PRESENT

- Anyone who has had a cardiac or respiratory arrest
- Those who are unconscious and unable to maintain an airway without assistance
- People from all age groups. Children usually have a respiratory problem first, for example, infection or foreign body obstruction. Cardiac arrest may follow. Adults may have either a cardiac or respiratory arrest as the primary event.

CAUSATIVE FACTORS

- Ischaemic heart disease is the most common cause.
- Others include drowning, trauma, substance overdose, hypothermia, hypovolaemia, anaphylaxis and hypoxia.

GENERAL AIMS OF EMERGENCY AID

- Maintain safety of rescuer and victim at all times, for example, by diverting traffic or by disconnecting the electrical source from the victim of electrocution before approaching him or her.
- Be able to diagnose a cardiac or respiratory arrest, assess the situation and start life support manoeuvres
- Maintain patient's oxygenation and perfusion by artifical methods until help arrives.

ASSESSMENT OF THE UNCONSCIOUS PERSON

- The new Resuscitation Council guidelines emphasise the need for a quick, full assessment of the patient first. If there is no one else to call an ambulance, the rescuer should leave the patient to call for help before starting treatment (except in the case of respiratory arrest). This is in order to get a defibrillator to the arrest victim as quickly as possible. It has now been shown that in most cases a defibrillator is the sole means of restarting the arrested heart.
- Check whether the patient is unconscious. Ask him or her loudly, 'Are you all right?' and shake gently by the shoulders (unless cervical spine injury is suspected). If the person does not respond, proceed with basic life support manoeuvres.

CLEARING THE AIRWAY

- The three commonest obstructions are false teeth, vomit and the tongue.
- If person has well-fitting dentures, leave them in place. If they are loose or he or she has a gum shield or bridge that poses a threat to the airway, remove them.

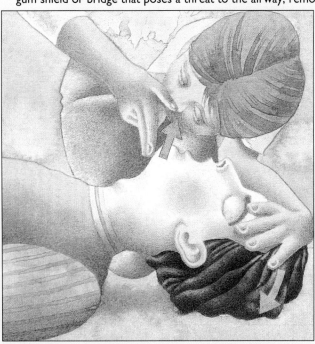

- If there is vomit, turn the head to the side and finger-sweep the vomit out of the mouth. This avoids aspiration.
- In the deeply unconscious patient lying supine the tongue will fall to the back of the hypopharynx and obstruct the airway. Rectify this by tilting the head back while lifting the chin.
- *Where there is evidence of trauma above the level of the clavicle it indicates a risk of cervical spine injury. These patients should not be moved except as a last resort or if their condition will be made worse by not moving them, that is, if they start to vomit while supine and unconscious.*

RE

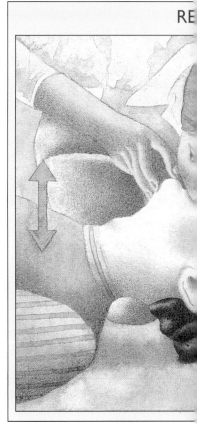

RE-ESTABLISHING THE PULSE

- After checking breathing, check the patient's carotid pulse. Feel this for five seconds. If there is a pulse, act as above.
- If the patient has no pulse, an ambulance should be summoned. Say that the patient's heart has stopped.
- Start ventilating and compressing: alternate two ventilations with 15 compressions`.
- Place the heel of one hand on the lower third of the sternum, two to three finger breadths away from the xiphisternum (this reduces the risk of gastric compression).
- Place your second hand flat on the back of the first and interlink your fingers to ensure they do not put pressure either side of the sternum. Careful hand placement reduces the incidence of rib breakage.
- Keep your elbows straight and your shoulders above your wrists. Your arms should be perpendicular to the patient's chest. This ensures that the massage relies on the weight of your thorax rather than muscular power which would quickly tire you.
- Your rate of compressions should be 80–100 a minute. This is to maximise coronary artery perfusion pressure during cardiac massage.
- If the patient is on a sprung bed, it is best to lie him or her on the floor if this can be done without risk.
- After basic full life support has been initiated following cardiac arrest, the pulse should not be rechecked unless the patient attempts a breath or makes a movement. Every five seconds spent checking the pulse is time without the compressions and ventilations which are vital to the patient.

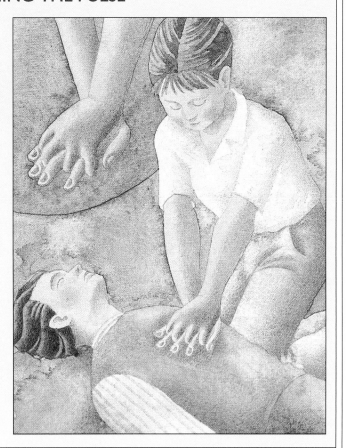

ABLISHING BREATHING

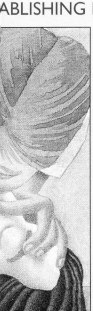

- Assess whether the patient is breathing by simultaneously looking for chest movement and listening for breath sounds. Do this for five seconds. Also feel for the patient's breath on your cheek.
- If the patient is breathing, feel the carotid pulse and put the patient in the recovery position. The carotid pulse can be felt about an inch either side of the centre of the thyroid cartilage (Adam's apple).
- If the patient is *not* breathing, feel the pulse, get someone to call an ambulance and state that the patient has stopped breathing.
- The patient should be given 10 artificial ventilations by mouth-to-mouth resuscitation, pocket mask or other ventilation device. The ventilations should be given slowly (10–12 per minute) and not too aggressively. Watch for the rising of the chest to indicate effectiveness.
- If you are on your own, give 10 artificial ventilations then leave patient and get help. On returning, support patient with ventilations alone, rechecking the pulse every 10 breaths. Maintain this until help arrives.

NOW YOU SHOULD BE ABLE TO:

- Adhere to the latest European Resuscitation Council guidelines for life support following a respiratory or cardiac arrest
- Understand the rationale for the manoeuvres and treatment given to the patient who has suffered a cardiopulmonary arrest
- Appreciate the importance of updating yourself in basic life support skills on a regular basis.

FURTHER READING
European Resuscitation Council Basic Life Support Working Group. Guidelines for basic life support. *British Medical Journal* 1993; **306**: 1587–1589.
Evans, T.R. (ed.). *ABC of Resuscitation* (2nd edn). London: British Medical Journal, 1990.
Royal College of Physicians. Resuscitation from cardiopulmonary arrest: training and organisation. *Journal of the Royal College of Physicians of London* 1987; **21**: 3, 2–8.
Wynne, G., Revival techniques. *Nursing Times* 1993; **89**: 11, 26–31.

INFORMATION
Information on basic life support courses and videos are available from local branches of the Red Cross, the St John Ambulance Association, the ambulance service or the resuscitation training officer at your local general hospital.

Petronelle Prior-Willeard, RGN, is resuscitation training officer, Royal Berkshire and Battle Hospital NHS Trust, Reading

BLADDER LAVAGE

- Bladder lavage is the washing out of the bladder with a sterile fluid, which may or may not include dissolved medication.
- Bladder irrigation refers to the continuous washing out of the bladder using a three-way catheter.

INDICATIONS FOR LAVAGE

- Lavage may help clear an obstructed catheter.
- The procedure can remove a potential source of future obstruction such as sediment from infection (for example, pus) or blood. Calcium and magnesium salts may also precipitate out of solution, forming a residue (struvite) which may obstruct a catheter.
- Note that cleansing the bladder with urinary disinfectants or antibiotics in cases of urinary infections is of dubious value and may be counter-productive.
- It should be remembered that urinary tract infections are very common and that catheterisation increases the incidence significantly. The catheter provides a route for micro-organisms to get into the bladder from where they may ascend to infect the renal system.

ADVANTAGES OF BLADDER WASH-OUTS

- Bladder wash-outs may help prevent or treat catheter obstruction.
- Sterile isotonic normal saline may be used and is widely available, although commercial preparations are often prescribed for community patients.

DISADVANTAGES OF BLADDER WASH-OUTS

- Regular bladder wash-outs may lead to infection with resistant organisms which results in higher rates of infection.
- There is no good evidence to believe that intermittent bladder wash-outs will prevent or remove urinary tract infection in catheterised individuals.
- The closed drainage system must be interrupted to carry out lavage. The single most important way to prevent infection entering via a catheter is to maintain a closed system.
- Because of these factors the procedure should only be carried out in the presence of a specific indication. This will usually be related to potential or actual obstruction.

- Gaining patient cooperation and maintenance of dignity are essential. The overall condition of the patient must be considered throughout the procedure.
- Aseptic technique must be maintained.
- All equipment should be assembled on a table or a tray.
- A sterile field is prepared using a dressing pack and the solution prepared in one of the foil bowls or jugs. If the solution is not going to be used at once it should be kept covered with a sterile paper towel. The solution should be as near body temperature as possible.
- Hands should be washed and sterile gloves put on.
- A sterile towel should be placed beneath the junction of the catheter and the drainage tube. The drainage tube may be clamped if necessary and then disconnected. The area around the end of the catheter should be cleaned and dried using a cleansing solution. This will help to remove surface organisms and so make their transfer into the lumen of the catheter less likely.
- The lavage solution should be drawn up into the bladder syringe, any air ejected and the syringe inserted into the end of the catheter. If a pre-prepared commercial preparation is employed this may be inserted directly into the catheter.
- Fifty to sixty millilitres of solution should be instilled gently into the bladder.

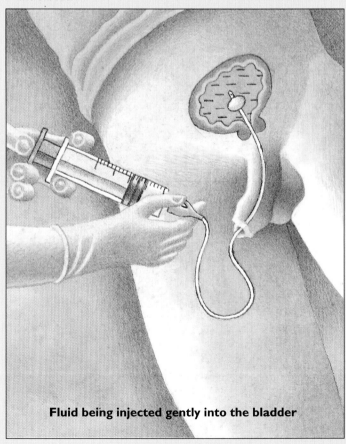

Fluid being injected gently into the bladder

...URE

- The syringe should be removed and the contents allowed to drain out naturally into the second sterile receiver. If the solution does not drain, very gentle aspiration may be applied using the bladder syringe. The introduction and drainage of solution is repeated until the returning solution is clear and any obstructions have been removed.
- If the solution is to be retained in the bladder the catheter should be spigoted. Manufacturers do not recommend clamping the catheter. The time should be noted so that the fluid can be retained for the prescribed period. When continuous drainage is to be resumed, a new tube and bag unit should be connected and any residual fluid allowed to drain. The system should not be left 'open' at any time as this will allow the entry of potentially harmful organisms.
- The volume of drained fluid should be measured and compared with the volume injected.
- All equipment should be hygienically disposed of.
- The patient should be advised to drink plenty of fluids. This keeps the urine dilute, so reducing precipitation, and promotes the flushing-out effect of potential pathogens.
- Mobility should be encouraged. Immobility will promote bony demineralisation and increase precipitation, which may obstruct the catheter.

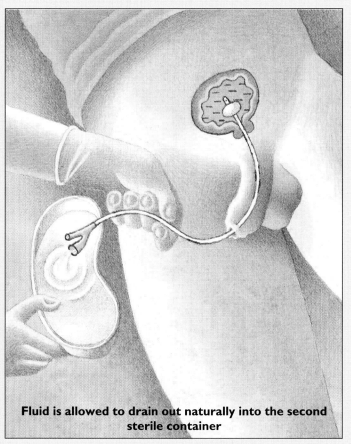

Fluid is allowed to drain out naturally into the second sterile container

EQUIPMENT REQUIRED

- A 50–60 ml bladder syringe
- Sterile dressing pack
- Sterile gloves
- Two sterile foil bowls or jugs
- Cleansing fluid
- Sterile spigot and new catheter drainage bag
- Sterile solution for lavage
- A clamp for the drainage tube
- Clinical waste bag

SELECTION OF LAVAGE SOLUTION

- Some bactericidal agents take time to have an effect. Noxythiolin (Noxyflex), now rarely used, for instance, is effective only if in contact with infected urine for two hours.[1] This means that such agents are often used incorrectly, giving no clinical benefit.
- Chlorhexidine (0.02%) can lead to selection of resistant bacterial strains, making future infections harder to treat. In addition, bladder erosion and haematuria may occur.[2]
- Chemical additives such as chlorhexidine and noxythiolin in lavage fluids can increase the number of bladder cells found in the drainage.[3] Bladder cell exfoliation also occurs with saline wash-outs, so the damage caused to the bladder lining is probably largely associated with physical damage caused by the procedure.
- Various other solutions including commercial preparations have been recommended for bladder wash-outs, such as mandelic acid 1% and citric acid 3.23% to combat catheter crystallisation.[4]

YOU SHOULD NOW BE AWARE OF:

- The indications for bladder wash-outs
- The complications associated with wash-outs
- The equipment necessary and the need for aseptic technique
- The general care of a patient with an indwelling catheter.

REFERENCES
[1] Kennedy, A. Trial of a new bladder wash-out system. *Nursing Times* 1984; 80: 46, 48–51.
[2] Pritchard, A.P. *Royal Marsden Hospital Manual of Clinical Nursing Procedures.* Oxford: Blackwell, 1992.
[3] Elliott, T. Disadvantages of bladder irrigation. *Nursing Times* 1990; 86: 4, 52.
[4] Flack, S. Finding the best solution. *Nursing Times* 1993; 89: 11, 68–74.

John Campbell, BA, RMN, RGN, DipN, CertEd, is nurse tutor, Lakeland College, Cumberland Infirmary, Carlisle

For male catheterisation, see page 20

TRACHEOSTOMIES

INDICATIONS

A tracheostomy is an artificial opening made into the trachea through the anterior wall below the crico-thyroid. Patency is ensured by the insertion of a curved tube of metal or plastic. Either permanent or temporary, this procedure ensures that a patent airway is maintained and allows removal of bronchial secretions.

A tracheostomy is indicated:

▨ Following surgery where normal respirations are compromised, for example, after laryngectomy.

It is important to remember that not all patients have a tracheostomy following laryngectomy. Some patients might only have a stoma opening without a tracheostomy tube being *in situ*.

▨ Neuromotor deficiency, for example, myasthenia or motor neurone disease

▨ Trauma to the mouth or upper airway

▨ In severe respiratory embarrassment where a tracheostomy is needed for respiratory support.

POINTS FOR CONSIDERATION

▨ The overriding concern is always the maintenance of tracheostomy patency — asphyxiation may occur if this is compromised. Blockage can occur if the tube becomes obstructed with a mucus clot or debris.

▨ Air inspired via a tracheostomy is not warmed, moistened or filtered, so each of these factors should be taken into consideration. In summer a small mesh may be worn over the opening to prevent inhalation of insects.

▨ Patient independence should be maximised, with specific training given for self-care. Partners and carers may also play an important role in tracheostomy care and maintenance.

▨ Support should be given and all carers should understand the frustrations that may result from the inability to speak normally. Time must be taken to communicate effectively.

▨ Mouth care should be provided to maintain oral hygiene.

▨ Water must not be allowed to enter the trachea. Patients should avoid swimming, and bathe rather than shower; lying down in the bath should be discouraged. It should not be assumed that patients will instinctively realise the danger of water entering the site.

CARE OF THE SITE

▨ As the stoma is a wound, the normal principles of asepsis and wound care apply. The area should be cleaned using sterile swabs and normal saline.

▨ A sterile keyhole dressing should be applied around the stoma and changed when it becomes wet; this will prevent excoriation and reduce the risk of infection.

▨ Gentle suction with a Yankeur catheter may be used around the stoma site to remove excess secretions.

▨ The tube should always be secured using tape tied in a square knot not a bow; alternatively, tracheostomy tube holders can be used.

ACCIDENTAL EXTUBATION

▨ It is advisable that a replacement tube and tracheal dilators are always to hand so that if extubation should occur the dilators may be used to maintain the patency of the airway prior to reintubation with a fresh tube. It should be noted, however, that long-term tracheostomies will be unlikely to close down immediately if the tube is, for example, coughed out.

▨ If the tube obstructs it is vital to replace it with a patent tube at once rather than wasting time trying to clear the existing tube.

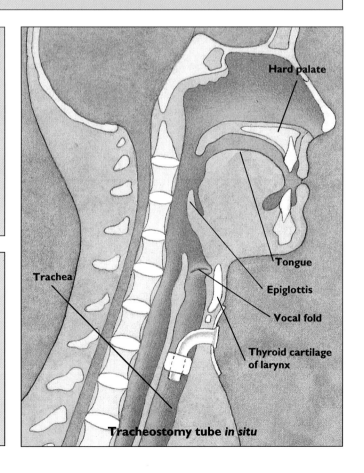

Hard palate

Tongue

Epiglottis

Vocal fold

Thyroid cartilage of larynx

Trachea

Tracheostomy tube *in situ*

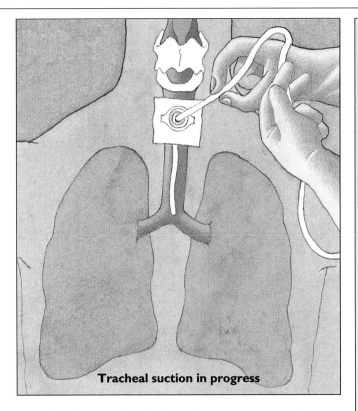

Tracheal suction in progress

EQUIPMENT REQUIRED FOR ROUTINE TUBE CHANGES

- Replacement tube and introducer
- 'Keyhole' dressing
- Sterile dressing pack
- Tracheostomy tape
- Sterile gloves
- Disposable plastic apron
- Barrier cream if indicated
- Sterile normal saline for cleansing
- Suction equipment
- Paper tissues
- Clinical waste bag

Note that: permanent tubes are usually made out of silver, as this is non-irritating. These may be cleaned and reused indefinitely. Some tubes are fitted with a flap valve to allow the user to talk. Portex temporary tubes often include an inflatable cuff.

PRINCIPLES FOR CARE

▪ Humidity

Several aids may increase air humidity. These include heated or unheated humidifiers and nebulisers. Room humidifiers are also available. Humidification of inhaled air keeps secretions non-viscous and easily mobilised; it also prevents the formation of thick, crusty secretions.

Stasis of secretions will increase the opportunity for infection. Systemic dehydration should be avoided as this will make chest secretions more tenacious.

▪ Physiotherapy

General whole body mobility should be promoted. If this is not possible, there should be frequent positional change and turning. Deep breathing should be encouraged and chest physiotherapy will encourage expectoration. Visits by a community physiotherapist may be arranged.

▪ Suction

Suction is used when the patient's 'cough' is ineffective or when secretions are too viscous for efficient expectoration. It is important to use the correct catheter size. Use of a large diameter catheter will cause irritation while a narrow lumen will not allow the passage of thick secretions — the catheter diameter should not exceed half the diameter of the tracheostomy tube. If the patient is mechanically ventilated he or she should be pre-oxygenated before suction to prevent possible hypoxia. A suction control unit may be placed between the catheter and the suction tubing and the suction machine set at the appropriate level.

A clean, fresh, disposable glove and a sterile catheter should be used for every insertion into the trachea. The catheter should be inserted no further than the carina, that is, it should not enter either of the main bronchi. The patient should be asked to take a breath as the catheter is inserted down the trachea. Suction is not applied during the insertion of the catheter. Once it is in place, suction is applied as the catheter is withdrawn in order to clear the tube's lumen of excess secretions. The patient may breathe out as the catheter is withdrawn. Suction should be limited to approximately 15 seconds in order not to interfere with normal breathing. Secretions should be observed for colour, volume and viscosity. Secretion volume may increase as a result of any inflammatory process. Green or yellow secretions indicate bacterial infection. Careful observation of the patient's overall condition throughout the procedure is essential as distress could be caused by compromising respirations.

NOW YOU SHOULD BE AWARE OF:

- The main principles for care of tracheostomies
- Techniques for tracheal suction
- The equipment required for tracheostomy tube changes and what to do in the event of accidental extubation or tube blockage.

FURTHER READING
Agnes, E.S. *Ear Nose and Throat Nursing* (6th edn). London: Baillière Tindall, 1983.
Freud, R.H. *Principles of Head and Neck Surgery*. New York: Appleton-Century-Croft, 1979.
Harris, R.B., Hyman, R.B. Clean versus sterile tracheostomy care and level of pulmonary infection. *Nursing Research* 1983; **33**: 2, 80–85.
Pritchard, A. P., Mallet, J. (Eds). *Royal Marsden Hospital Manual of Clinical Nursing Procedures*. Oxford: Blackwell, 1992.

John Campbell, BA, RMN, RGN, DipN, CertEd, is a nurse tutor, Lakeland College, Cumberland Infirmary, Cumberland

UNDERTAKING URINALYSIS

WHO WILL PRESENT

A urinalysis may be required during the following consultations:
- Routine care from GP, practice or district nurse
- Medical examinations for insurance
- Occupational health screenings
- Annual screenings of the over 75s
- Well-woman/man clinics
- Screenings of school children
- Antenatal testing
- Pre-surgery screenings.

COLLECTING A SPECIMEN

- Ideally, a clean mid-stream urine (MSU) specimen will be collected in a wide-mouthed container with a lid. Both should be scrupulously clean and uncontaminated from previous contents or cleaning fluids.
- The client must wash his/her hands and settle over the toilet. The external genitalia should be wiped using cotton wool or toilet tissue and tap water. Uncircumcised males should retract the foreskin and clean around glans and meatus. Females should clean from front to rear under the labia.
- Clients should pass a small amount of urine into the toilet to flush the urethra, and then pass the main stream into the collection container, ensuring this does not touch the external genitalia. The client should then stop and complete the stream into the toilet.
- The specimen should be tested while fresh and should not be allowed to stand.
- Elderly or disabled clients may need assistance. Translated instructions are needed for clients who do not speak English.

POTENTIAL CAUSES OF HAEMATURIA

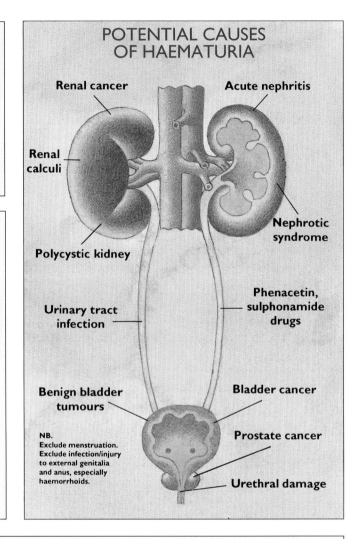

- Renal cancer
- Acute nephritis
- Renal calculi
- Nephrotic syndrome
- Polycystic kidney
- Phenacetin, sulphonamide drugs
- Urinary tract infection
- Benign bladder tumours
- Bladder cancer
- Prostate cancer
- Urethral damage

NB.
Exclude menstruation.
Exclude infection/injury to external genitalia and anus, especially haemorrhoids.

TESTING THE SPECIMEN

- Multistix dry-chemistry reagent strips have chemical pads. Each pad is used to detect a single analyte using colour change to indicate the results.
- Check the expiry date and ensure the bottle is closed tightly after use and stored in cool, dry conditions, as humidity and extremes of temperature cause deterioration.
- Do not touch the reagent pads. Using gloves, immerse the strip fully into the specimen for one to two seconds, ensuring all pads are covered. Remove and gently tap on the side of container to remove excess urine.
- Hold strip horizontally to prevent mixing of reagents and check each pad carefully against the colour chart printed on the bottle or on bench readers that can be obtained from Bayer Diagnostics.

- It is important to adhere to the testing times specified in the manufacturer's instructions, especially those with quantitative results.
- Test one patient's specimen at a time — never dip, leave and return.
- If you suspect a false positive result caused by an inappropriate container, wrong method of collection or a delay in testing, then request that a repeat specimen is collected in a sterile container and, if necessary, supervise the collection.
- Record all the results in the client's notes.
- Inform the doctor of any abnormal findings. There should be a protocol to establish whether any further tests and/or medical examinations are necessary.

CLINICAL SIGNIFICANCE AND ACTION

THE SPECIFIC GRAVITY

The specific gravity (SG) reflects the concentration of urine, bodily hydration, concentration of solutes in urine and functioning of the kidneys. Normal SG is 1.002 –1.035.

Decreased SG (dilute) will occur in clients with nephritis, diabetes insipidus or excess fluid intake.

Increased SG (concentrated) is associated with vomiting, diarrhoea, fever, excess sweating and diminished fluid intake.

THE NORMAL pH

Normal pH of urine is 4.5–8. The pH reflects the acid-base balance.

A low pH (acidity) occurs in clients with metabolic acidosis, diabetic ketoacidosis, diarrhoea, dehydration, starvation, fever and certain infections.

A high pH (alkalinity) occurs in clients with renal failure, vomiting, metabolic alkalosis and certain infections.

- *Action:* If a high reading is found, indicating stale urine, a fresh sample should be taken.

Note: SG and pH give supportive information to the other reagent tests.

PROTEIN

A positive protein result will occur in clients with infection, hypertension, renal disease, gout, amyloidosis, toxaemia (in pregnant women) or possibly in clients who have been standing for some time before giving the specimen.

- *Action:*
  — Test a repeat specimen and check for nitrates and leucocytes
  — Check specimen and client for signs of urinary tract infection
  — Check blood pressure; ask whether client has had headaches
  — Look for swollen hands, ankles, puffy face.
- *Follow-up:* asymptomatic proteinuria may be the first indicator of renal disease. MSU for culture and sensitivity or, in the absence of infection, MSU for protein estimation.

GLUCOSE

A positive test for glucose will occur in clients with a lowered renal threshold (in elderly and pregnant clients) or diabetes mellitus

- *Action:*
  — Continued observation of elderly people and pregnant women
  — Check for signs of diabetes, such as increased thirst, weight loss, tiredness, polyuria, genital pruritis, skin infections, boils
  — Test for ketones.

- *Follow-up:* a capillary sample should be tested on a blood glucose strip or a laboratory test should be undertaken for random blood glucose estimation.

KETONES

In the absence of usable glucose, the body will break down fat, and the by-product, ketones, are excreted in the urine. A positive result will occur in clients with diabetic ketoacidosis, vomiting, diarrhoea, fever or those on a low carbohydrate diet or suffering from starvation or anorexia.

- *Action:*
  — Smell specimen for acetone
  — Test for glucose
  — Check for symptoms of diabetes
  — Ask about recent illness and diet.
- *Follow-up:* urgent referral in the case of uncontrolled or new diabetes.

BILIRUBIN AND UROBILINOGEN

Bile pigments may be found in the urine where there is an obstruction of their outlet into the gut. A positive test will occur in clients with obstruction/abnormality in liver or biliary system, gall stones, cholecystitis, cancer of the head of the pancreas, cirrhosis or hepatitis, whether viral or drug-induced — for example, through taking chlorpromazine.

- *Action:*
  — Observe for yellow discoloration of skin and eyes
  — Ask about general health, abdominal pains or discomfort, nausea, drug therapy, alcohol intake.
- *Follow-up:* take a blood sample for liver function tests, urea, electrolytes and full blood count.

BLOOD

Seen as frank blood or haemolysed cells releasing their pigments (see 'Potential Causes of Haematuria', left).

- *Action:*
  — Check specimen and client for signs of urinary tract infection
  — Ask about drug therapy and presence of any pains.
- *Follow-up:* MSU to laboratory for analysis.

NITRATES AND LEUCOCYTES

Both are indicative of urinary tract infection (UTI).

- *Action:*
  — Check sample for smell, cloudiness, particles
  — Check specimen for blood and protein
  — Ask about symptoms of UTI: frequency of, or burning, on micturition; loin pain, fever. A high percentage of UTIs are silent and asymptomatic, yet they are still damaging to the renal system and need urgent treatment.
- *Follow-up:* MSU for culture of organisms and antibiotic sensitivity.

YOU SHOULD NOW FEEL COMPETENT TO:

- Examine an uncontaminated urine specimen
- Take appropriate action regarding any abnormal findings.

FURTHER READING
Newall, R.G. *Clinical Urinalysis.* Basingstoke: Bayer Diagnostics, 1990.

Irene Heywood Jones, SRN, RMN, ONC, DipN, RNT, is a nurse tutor in orthopaedics and elderly care and a freelance writer

REMOVAL OF SUTURES AND STAPLES

WHO WILL PRESENT?

■ Any patient following a surgical procedure or repair of trauma, who is considered ready to continue recovery at home and has community support arranged.

■ Patients who have had common orthopaedic operations such as menisectomy, hip and knee arthroplasty (joint replacement) and back surgery to correct prolapsed intervertebral disc. Also various operations on the hands and feet and occasionally the shoulder.

GENERAL POINTS OF CONSIDERATION

■ Discharge home will only be sanctioned once the multidisciplinary team is certain that the patient is generally well, is safely ambulant and has a sound, clean wound.

■ Certain individual circumstances may delay healing, such as diabetes, steroid therapy, obesity, malnutrition, anaemia, heart or lung disease, malignancy, jaundice, uraemia, stress, pre-existing infection in the wound site, peri- or post-operative infection, or if the person is frail and elderly.

■ It is predominantly elderly patients who have orthopaedic surgery.

■ The method of skin closure determines its removal. Ensure that the discharge information identifies the specific type of closure, so that you are prepared with the correct equipment. When in doubt, check with the ward staff.

WOUND ASSESSMENT AND MANAGEMENT

■ The discharge sheet should give an appropriate guide when to remove skin closures. These are arbitrary periods and the ultimate decision lies with the clinical discretion of the practitioner and the assessment of wound healing.

■ The surgeon may request the wound to remain covered with a commercial dressing or, more usually on discharge, will request it to be left free to the air. Some patients feel uneasy with an exposed wound and are happier if a light gauze dressing covers it for part of the day. This also prevents suture ends/beads/staples from catching on clothing.

■ Check the wound is healing as expected. Any wound infection will require systemic antibiotics to be prescribed by the GP. (It is routine in major invasive orthopaedic surgery, especially insertion of a prosthesis, for patients to be given antibiotic cover, on induction or with the premedication, plus an intramuscular/oral course.)

■ If individual sutures or staples are infected, these should be removed and this small area held firm with a proprietary adhesive skin closure while healing takes place.

■ Practitioners may decide to remove alternate sutures/staples initially to double-check the security of the wound, and then remove those remaining a day or two later.

■ Following removal of sutures/staples, any slight gaping of the wound, or suggestion of such, can be held secure with adhesive skin closures. Continue to monitor the patient until healing is complete.

REMOVAL O

There are several staple insertion/removal systems on the market and ideally removers should be matched with a compatible staple type. Do not use Michel clip removers on staples. These are far too heavy and unsuitable; they may snap the light staple bar and leave the prongs stranded inside the patient.

The procedure for staple removal is as follows:

■ Prepare the patient physically and psychologically.

■ Check the movement of the remover handles and alignment of the jaws, keeping it away from the patient's skin.

■ Insert both tips of the lower jaw under the staple bar, trying to avoid contact or pressure on the incision line.

■ Lift slightly, so the sides of the staple are perpendicular to the plane of the skin.

■ Gently squeeze the handles together. This brings the jaws together and frees the two prongs from the skin.

■ Lift the reformed staple straight up and discard.

■ Check the wound and apply adhesive skin closure to weak areas.

■ Settle the patient and dispose of equipment safely.

■ Skin clips, Michel and Kifa, have largely been superseded by stapling, but if these are used they are removed in the same way, using the appropriate clip remover.

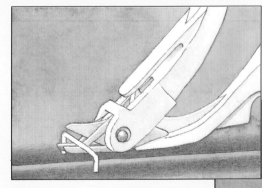

EQUIPMENT FOR REMOVAL OF SUTURES OR STAPLES

The nurse needs a sterile pack or individual items of the following:
- Stitch cutter or scissors, or appropriate staple remover
- Forceps or gloves
- Gauze
- Disposal bag
- Adhesive skin closures

SKIN STAPLES

There is a growing popularity in the use of metal staples as the choice for skin closure in neurosurgery, gynaecology, orthopaedics, general and vascular surgery, all types of minimal access surgery and selected trauma cases in A & E. The wound is managed in exactly the same way as a conventional sutured wound and the time scales for healing are the same. The advantages of skin staples include:
- The staples grasp only the superficial layer of skin, providing a secure hold in apposition, yet with less underlying tissue trauma than with suturing.
- The bar of the staple hovers above the incision line, so there is less likelihood of the cross hatching effect of sutures.

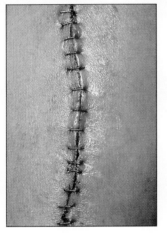

Patients sometimes complain of discomfort when staples are removed. Although this does not appear to be a great problem and is momentary, it is important that nurses warn the patient prior to staple removal that he or she may feel a slight stinging, nipping or pulling.

SKIN SUTURES AND THEIR REMOVAL

The practitioner is likely to encounter different methods of suturing, including conventional styles and some highly individual modifications by surgeons. There may also be a combination of alternating sutures and staples.

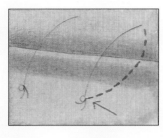

The procedure for suture removal is as follows:
- Prepare the patient physically and psychologically.
- The prevailing principle is always to avoid pulling the exposed, contaminated part of the suture through sterile tissue beneath the skin.
- Using forceps, hold firmly the knot or bead, apply slight traction to lift the suture material free from its bed and cut the suture close to the skin edge.
- Always pull the suture free towards the incision line rather than putting tension on the wound edges.
- If a fragment of suture material accidentally breaks loose and remains in the wound tissue it may set up irritation and infection, perhaps even leading to a sinus formation. However, it should soon work itself free to the surface of the skin and be easily removed. Warn the patient that this may occur if it seems a possibility.

NOW YOU SHOULD FEEL COMPETENT TO:

- Remove all types of sutures and staples that are encountered in your practice.

Irene Heywood Jones, SRN, RMN, ONC, DipN, RNT, is a nurse tutor in orthopaedics and elderly care at St Vincents Hospital, Pinner, and a freelance writer

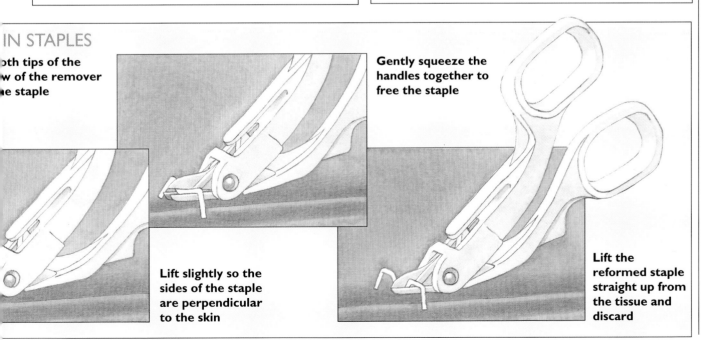

IN STAPLES

oth tips of the
w of the remover
e staple

Lift slightly so the sides of the staple are perpendicular to the skin

Gently squeeze the handles together to free the staple

Lift the reformed staple straight up from the tissue and discard

WHEN WILL A MALE CATHETER BE REQUIRED?

There are many indications for inserting a urinary catheter into the male bladder, although only two are generally applicable to long-term catheterisation in the community:
■ To bypass an obstruction
■ To relieve incontinence when no other means is practicable.[1]

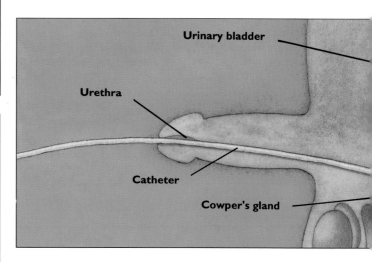

Urinary bladder

Urethra

Catheter

Cowper's gland

GENERAL CONSIDERATIONS

■ Passing a male catheter may not be part of a nurse's basic training and any nurse carrying out this procedure must ensure that she has undertaken the appropriate training. This article is designed to help nurses increase their awareness of this procedure, not teach students how to catheterise.
■ Acute retention of urine is a urological emergency for which the patient will require a medical assessment, therefore a clinician may be the best person to undertake the procedure. Such patients may also be difficult to catheterise.
■ Controversy exists as to whether a female nurse should undertake male catheterisation,[2] but it does allow the female nurse to undertake the full range of nursing care for the patient as well as eliminating unnecessary hospitalisation.
■ Sexuality should be considered with long-term catheterisation and patients may need advice and support as well as practical guidance on the subject. Catheters may be taped back along the penis once an erection is achieved to enable intercourse to take place.[3] However, this can cause trauma and urethral stricture formation.[4] For the sexually active it may be more appropriate to consider intermittent catheterisation or a supra-pubic catheter.

INSERTING AN INDWELLIN

■ The catheter should be passed using a strict aseptic technique and using the correct size of catheter and balloon for the patient.[1]
■ Assemble the equipment and make sure the bed is protected. The patient should be supine with the legs extended. Ensure privacy.
■ Open the packs using an aseptic technique. Wash hands and put on sterile gloves.
■ Place sterile towels across the patient's thighs and pubic region to ensure a sterile working field. Place the receiver between the legs.
■ Wrap sterile gauze around the penis and retract the foreskin. Cleanse the glans penis with either sterile water, sodium chloride 0.9% or antiseptic solution using forceps.
■ Insert the nozzle of the lubrication gel into the urethral opening and squeeze the gel into the urethra. Lubrication will reduce trauma and the local anaesthetic will minimise discomfort (see below).

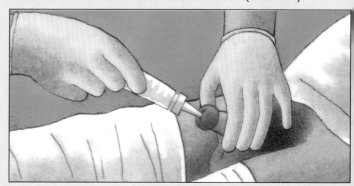

■ Grasp the penis shaft and raise until almost fully extended. Maintain this position until the catheter is passed — this will straighten the urethra and facilitate catheterisation.
■ Insert the tip of the catheter into the urethra and slowly advance the catheter until 20cm is passed. Urine should start to flow. Some resistance may be felt if there is spasm of the external sphincter. By increasing traction on the penis and applying gentle pressure this should be resolved.[1] Encouraging the patient to cough at this point may also ease passage of the catheter. Never force the catheter as this exerts undue trauma (see top right).

CATHETER SELECTION

For long-term catheter use (over two weeks) a silicone, silicone elastometer-coated latex or hydrogel-coated latex catheter should be used.
■ There is evidence from *in vitro* studies and clinical usage[5–7] to suggest that a hydrogel-coated latex catheter has better encrustation resistance than others, can be left *in situ* longer and is non-cytotoxic.
■ Catheters should be the smallest size capable of providing drainage. Sizes over 18 Ch should be questioned.
■ Balloon size should be 10ml.[8] A 30ml balloon will sit higher in the bladder and may cause irritation of the bladder trigone, leading to spasm and leaking of urine.[4]

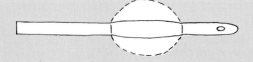

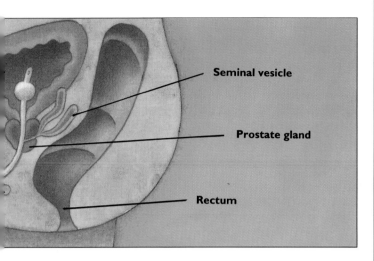

Seminal vesicle

Prostate gland

Rectum

PROBLEMS ASSOCIATED WITH LONG-TERM CATHETERISATION

■ Trauma from catheter insertion is the most common reason for urethral stricture formation. Trauma results from using a catheter too large, forcing the catheter on insertion or inflating the balloon in the urethra instead of the bladder. Traumatic removal with the balloon inflated also leads to stricture formation.

■ Too large a catheter may obstruct the para-urethral ducts, allowing accumulated bacteria to form an abcess. This could lead to formation of a cutaneous fistula as erosion of healthy tissue around the urethra develops. Prostatitis, prostatic abcess and epididymitis may also occur for the same reason.

■ Too large a catheter or balloon may cause traction on the bladder neck, leading to necrosis.[3] Pressure sores can also occur around the meatus if cleansing is inadequate and care not taken.

■ If the catheter has a non-deflating balloon because the inflating/deflation channel is sticking, the water can usually be aspirated from the inflation arm just above the valve.[10] Never cut off the end of the inflation channel to try to release the water. Always refer the patient to hospital.

■ Bacteriuria as a result of long-term catheterisation is virtually unavoidable but usually asymptomatic.[3] Closed urine drainage systems reduce the incidence of urinary tract infection and should be encouraged at all times.

HETER IN A MALE PATIENT

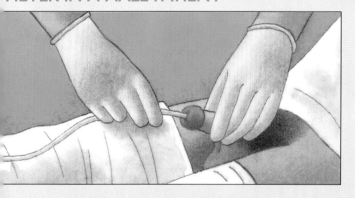

■ Ensure the catheter is in the bladder before inflating the balloon with sterile water, according to the manufacturer's instructions. Inadvertent inflation in the urethra will cause pain (see below).

■ Attach the catheter to a sterile drainage bag and reduce and reposition the foreskin. Failure to pull the foreskin back over the glans will result in paraphimosis.

■ Ensure the catheter bag is well supported on the leg to prevent traction on the catheter.

■ Manufacturers of catheters recommend that, when catheters are intended for long-term use, they should be replaced after a maximum of 12 weeks.[9]

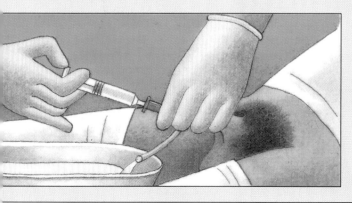

YOU SHOULD NOW BE AWARE OF:

■ The procedures involved in passing a male catheter
■ The complications that can result from male catheterisation.

REFERENCES
[1] Pritchard, A.P., David, J.A. *Royal Marsden Hospital Manual of Clinical Nursing Procedures* (2nd edn). London: Harper and Row, 1988.
[2] Pomfret, I. Generalist or specialist plumber. *Journal of District Nursing* 1985; **3:** 11, 24.
[3] Britton, P. M., Wright, E. S. Nursing care of catheterised patients. *Professional Nurse* 1990; **5:** 231–234.
[4] Norton, C. *Nursing for Continence.* Beaconsfield: Beaconsfield Publishers, 1986.
[5] Cox, A. J., Hukins, D.W.L., Millington, R . S. et al. Resistance of catheters coated with a modified hydrogel to encrustation during *in vitro* test. *Urological Research* 1989; **17:** 6, 353–356.
[6] Bull, E., Chilton, C. P., Gould, C.A.L. et al. A single-blind randomised, parallel group comparison of the Bard Biocath Catheter with a silicone elastomer-coated catheter: a community study. *British Journal of Urology* 1991; **68:** 4, 394–399.
[7] Nancy, J.N., Delahunt, B. Toxicity study of first and second generation hydrogel-coated latex urinary catheters. *British Journal of Urology* 1991; **67:** 3, 314–316.
[8] Health Care Standards Policy Committee. *Urological Catheters: Parts 1 and 2* (BS 1695). London: British Standards Institution, 1990.
[9] Roe, B., Brockenhurst, J.C. Study of patients with indwelling catheters. *Journal of Advanced Nursing* 1987; **12:** 713–718.
[10] Bard. *Guidelines for the Management of the Catheterised Patient.* Crawley: Bard Ltd, 1984.

Sue Thomas, RGN, RM, DN, CPT, is professional officer of the District Nursing Association

WHO WILL PRESENT

Any patient discharged with a plaster of Paris cast, such as:
- Upper limb cast for fractures of the arm and wrist, notably the Colles' fracture
- Lower limb cast for fractures of the tibia or around the ankle joint
- Casts to provide support or rest for an injured or strained joint or plastering for a diabetic foot ulcer.

IMPORTANT POINTS

- Patients may have difficulty retaining the information given to them in A&E owing to shock, the effects of anaesthesia and pain or cognitive impairment in elderly people.
- Worries or complaints from patients about their cast or limb must never be ignored, as damage caused by an ill-fitting cast may be irreversible.
- Whenever in doubt about the safety of the limb or cast, always advise patients to return to A&E without delay.

BACKGROUND TO CARE: ACCIDENT AND EMERGENCY

- Reduction of a fracture and application of the plaster may be accomplished using a short general or regional anaesthetic, such as Bier's block for the arm.
- If there is a lot of swelling around the site of injury, either present or anticipated, the limb may be held initially in a backslab plaster secured with bandages which is completed to a full plaster of Paris cast later.
- The limb must be elevated to reduce swelling — that is, an arm should be held in a sling, a leg raised on supportive pillows or cushions.
- Before discharge the patient will be given verbal instructions about plaster care and observations and a written sheet for them to refer to.
- For pain relief patients will be recommended a proprietary over-the-counter oral analgesic such as paracetamol (it should not be for pain from too tight a plaster).
- Patients must be accompanied home or have transport arranged for them.
- Patients with a leg plaster may be admitted for a night or two. The affected limb should not be weight-bearing during the 72 hours while the plaster dries and perhaps for a further few weeks. Patients will be given a cast slipper or boot and a walking frame, crutches or stick to enable them to walk without putting pressure on the new plaster.
- The patient will be asked to return to the A&E department after 24 hours for a plaster check or sooner if they develop problems. However, if this is difficult, A&E staff may arrange for the plaster check to be carried out by a district nurse, practice nurse or GP.

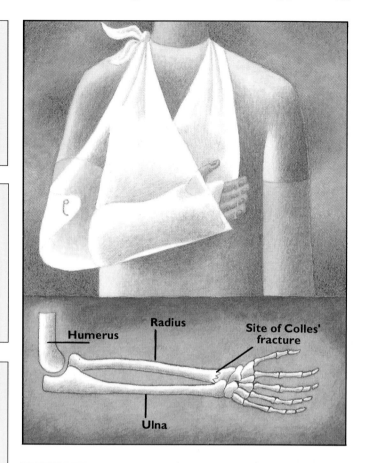

Humerus · Radius · Site of Colles' fracture · Ulna

MANAGING A NEW WET PLASTER

- A conventional plaster of Paris can take 24–72 hours to dry and harden completely, depending on the size and thickness, although with newer techniques drying may be faster.
- In the initial drying process, the chemical exothermic reaction of the plaster gives off heat, so the client will experience a warm sensation to the limb.
- To avoid indentations that may lead to plaster sores, handling of the plaster must be with the flat palms of the hands, not the fingertips. The client must not rest the cast on any firm edge of a table, chair or bed frame or knock it against furniture or a walking frame.
- The damp cast must be left exposed to facilitate drying. This must be achieved by evaporation from exposure to air. Artificial heat from a fire, heater or radiator must not be used as this will cause the plaster to crack.
- To absorb moisture it is advisable to take several firm pillows or cushions, cover these first with plastic bags or disposable bin liners for their protection, then apply cotton pillowcases or towels. Pillows must be turned to provide a dry patch for absorption and the position of the plastered limb changed to prevent a soggy spot from developing.

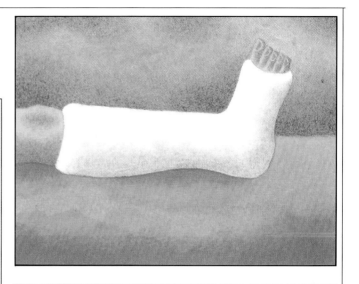

OBSERVING FOR DANGERS

- A plaster cast should fit closely to ensure that the fractured bone ends are held soundly together, yet not be so tight as to occlude blood vessels, press on nerves or cause excoriation of the skin. The final set cast will be firm and inflexible, with smooth edges.
- Swelling of the limb in response to injury is to be expected in the early days and can be a serious complication if it compromises the circulation and nerve supply to the limb. The limb must be maintained in an elevated position and the digits and unplastered joints mobilised. This will reduce the likelihood of swelling. The limb must not be allowed to hang down unless it is actively being used.
- Check for feeling, sensation and movement of the digits. A tingling or 'pins and needles' sensation indicates paraesthesia. Numbness indicates loss of sensation and nerve compression.
- The digits should feel warm, although they may be cool while the plaster is still damp or generally in a cold environment. Digits should look a healthy pink and, on applying pressure to the nailbed, this should blanch then reflush immediately. Impaired arterial circulation is indicated by blue, grey or white skin, delay in reflushing after blanching, marked swelling of the digits and pain on passive movement. Impaired venous return results in red, swollen, shiny digits. When clients are checking the warmth and colour of digits, tell them to compare them with those on the sound limb.
- Plaster casts are inclined to create an itching sensation. Clients must be firmly discouraged from inserting objects down the cast to scratch with (popular items are knitting needles, spoon handles and long-tailed combs), as these may damage the skin surface or cause infection. Development of a pressure sore is indicated by a blister-like, burning sensation initially, although pain subsides once the sore is established; the next stage will be a foul smell or discharge and perhaps staining of the cast which should be investigated.
- Exercise should be encouraged for all joints not encased in plaster, as these are prone to stiffening, particularly fingers, shoulders, elbows and knees, especially in elderly people. Active movements will maintain muscle strength and joint function, prevent atrophy and stiffness and help in later rehabilitation once the cast is removed. Clients with an arm in plaster should remove the arm from the sling frequently to put joints through their natural range of movements. Encourage use of the hand for everyday activities but keep it elevated when at rest. A leg at rest should be elevated to above the horizontal position.
- Clients should be advised to contact the hospital if their cast becomes cracked, loose, tight, stained or smelly or develops soft areas or ragged edges.

HOME MANAGEMENT FOR DAILY LIVING

- Many clients seeking advice will be elderly, infirm or handicapped in other ways, living alone and perhaps without access to transport or communication links.
- Clients may be made unsteady or incapacitated by the presence of any plaster, especially if the dominant arm is involved or they are managing on a frame or crutches. This may affect their ability to dress, shop, cook or clean.
- Once dry, the plaster must not get wet or it will disintegrate and fail to support the limb. Personal hygiene may pose a problem and use of a rubber glove or plastic bag can help protect the cast. Commercial covers are available but are expensive for brief use. If an elderly person is unsteady and in danger of falling while having a bath, recommend strip washes instead.
- Clients may need assistance from social services, meals on wheels, family or good neighbours.
- Clothing should preferably be loose and baggy with elasticated waists; jumpers, sweatshirts and tracksuits are ideal or old trousers split at the seams with Velcro attachments. Large socks, legwarmers and gloves may be worn to cover exposed digits.

YOU SHOULD NOW FEEL COMPETENT TO:

- Make reasoned observations and assess danger signs of plaster of Paris
- Provide sound advice to a client living with a plaster
- Know when to seek help from A & E staff.

FURTHER READING
Betts-Symonds, G.W. *Fracture: Care and Management for Students.* London: Macmillan, 1984.
Smith and Nephew. *A Practical Guide to Casting.* Hull: Smith and Nephew, 1991.

Irene Heywood Jones, SRN, RMN, ONC, DipN, RNT, is a nurse tutor in orthopaedics and elderly care at St Vincent's Hospital, Pinner, and a freelance writer